MW00510401

THE FiSH WHO WiSHED HE COULD EAT FRUIT

By Kathleen Stefancin, M.S., R.D.
Illustrated by Kirk Werner

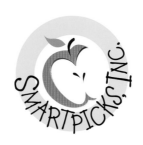

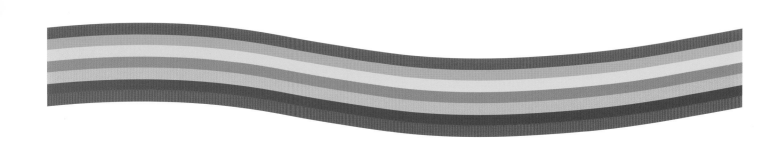

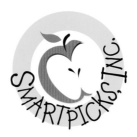

Smart Picks, Inc., P.O. Box 771440, Lakewood, Ohio 44107

Or visit:

www.smartpicks.com

ISBN 978-0-9764785-1-5

Library of Congress Control Number: 2006910314

Printing by Amica International, Inc., Seattle, Washington
First printing, January 2007

Printed in China

Book design, cover art and all illustrations by Kirk Werner

A sweet thanks to my dear friend Donna Drozda, for believing in me all these years. You are a tremendous inspiration!

—K.S.

Thanks to my Aunt Jean, for your enthusiastic support of my work!

—K.W.

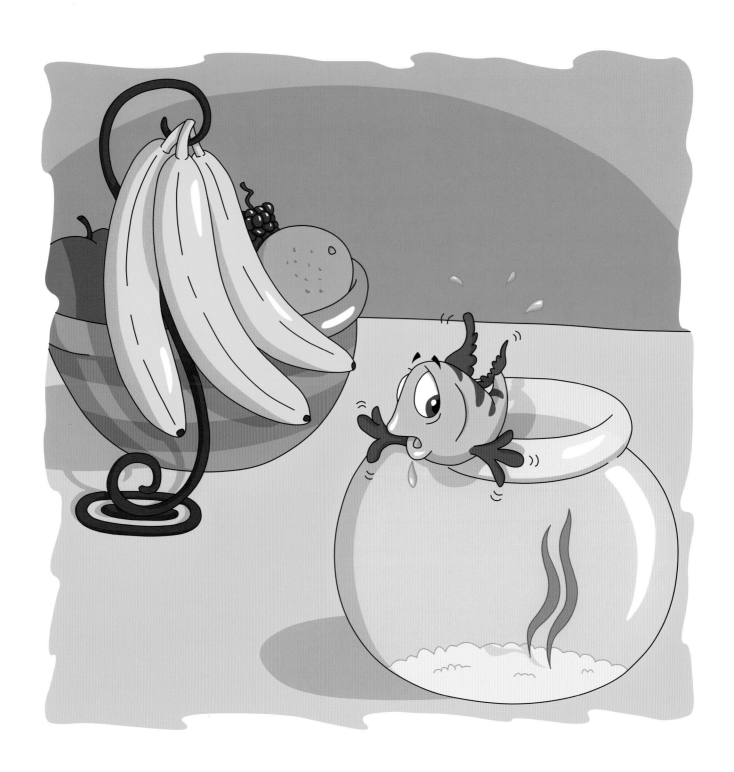

Theo almost fell out of his fish bowl
when he tried to reach the bananas
hanging from the banana tree.

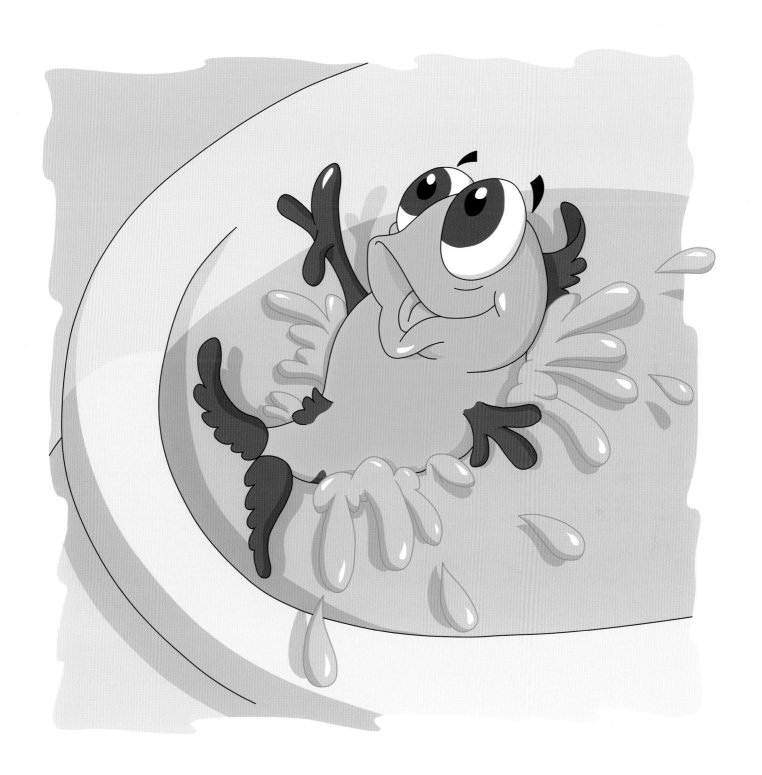

Plop!
Back into the water he went.
I almost got them, he thought.

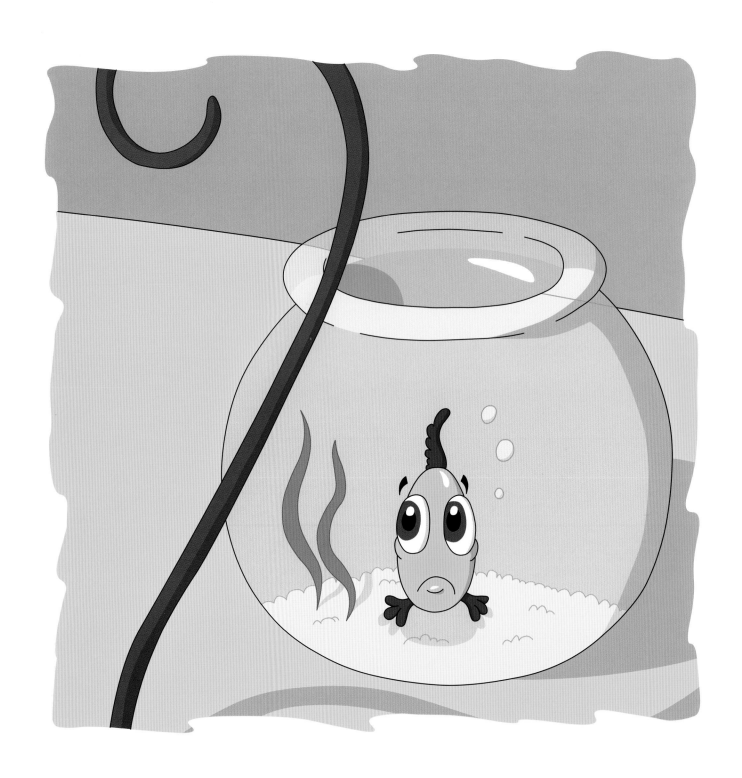

"Oh no, they're gone!"
Bananas didn't stay long on the banana tree.

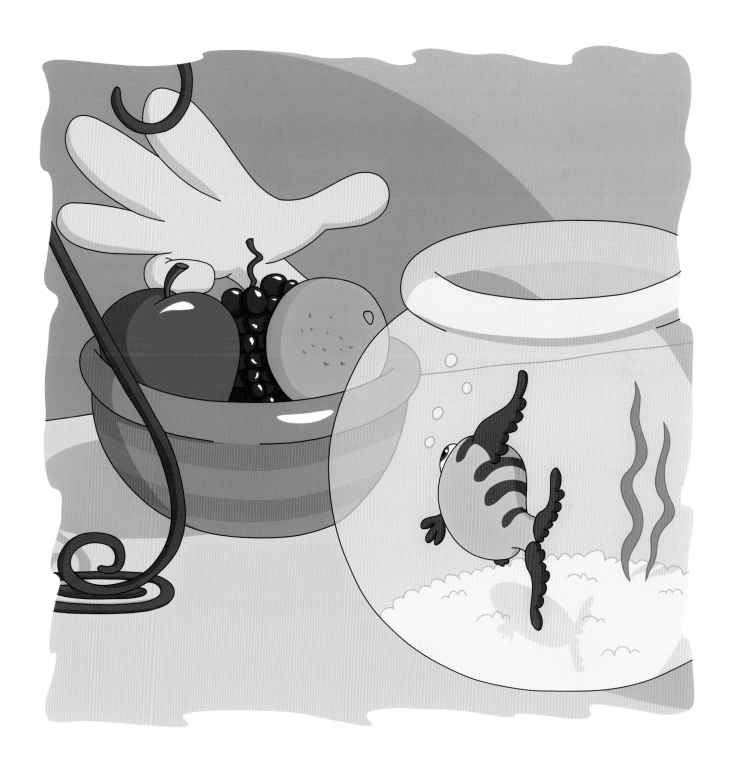

Neither did the red apples, oranges or purple grapes
in the dish right outside his fish bowl.

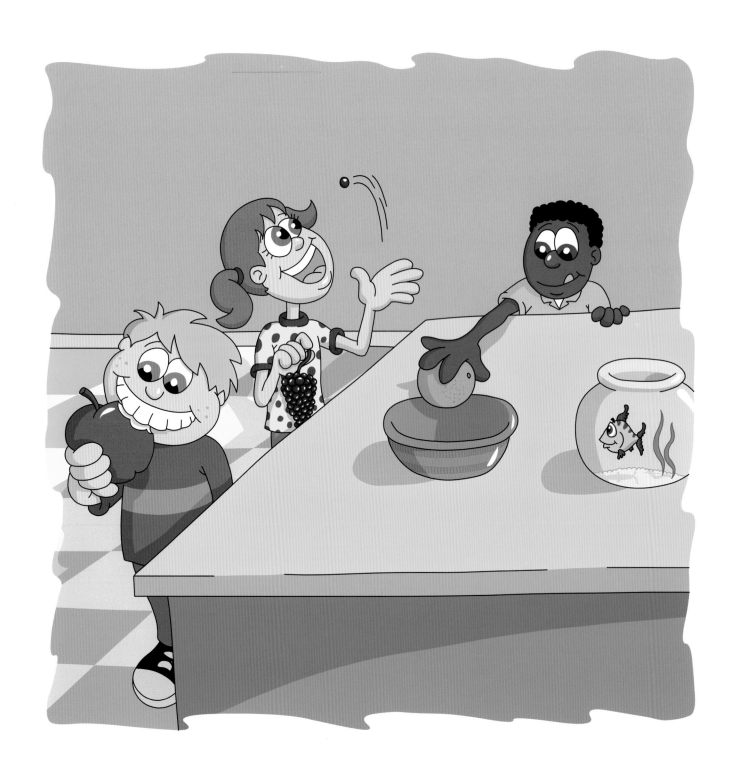

The children in the house were always eating the fruit
set out each day.

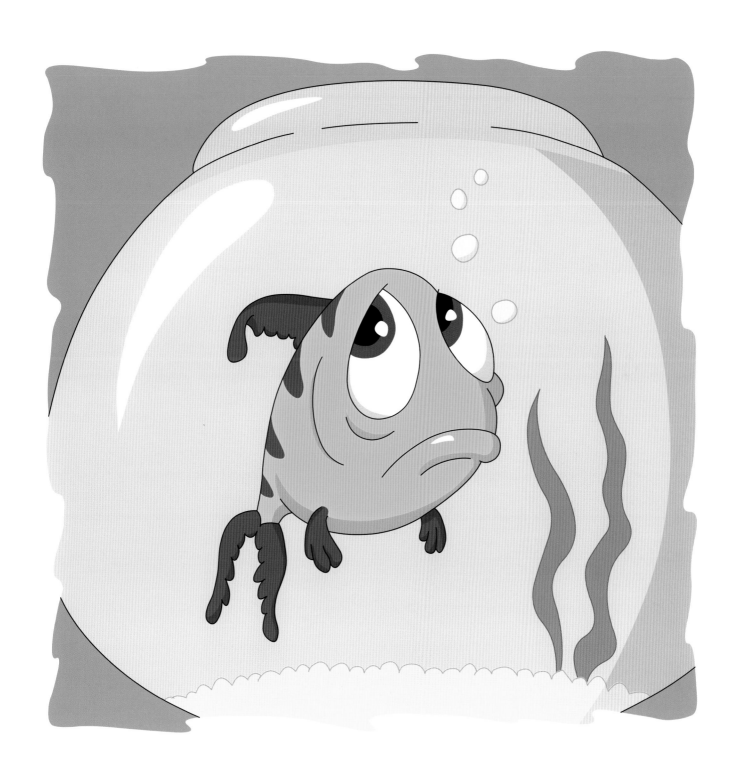

Theo wanted so badly to taste a piece of fruit.
"I'll try again tomorrow," he sighed.

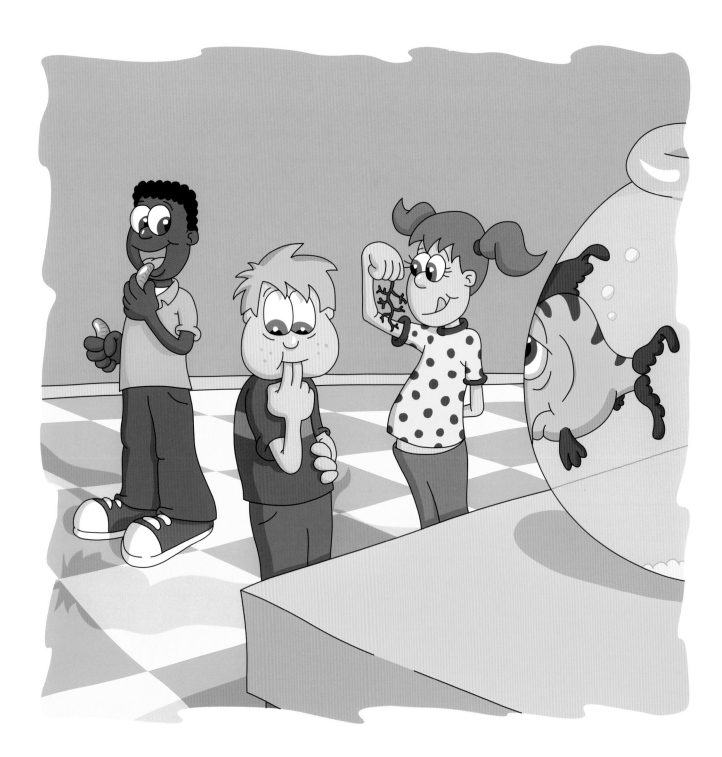

He stared out through the glass bowl, watching
the children smile as they ate every last bite.

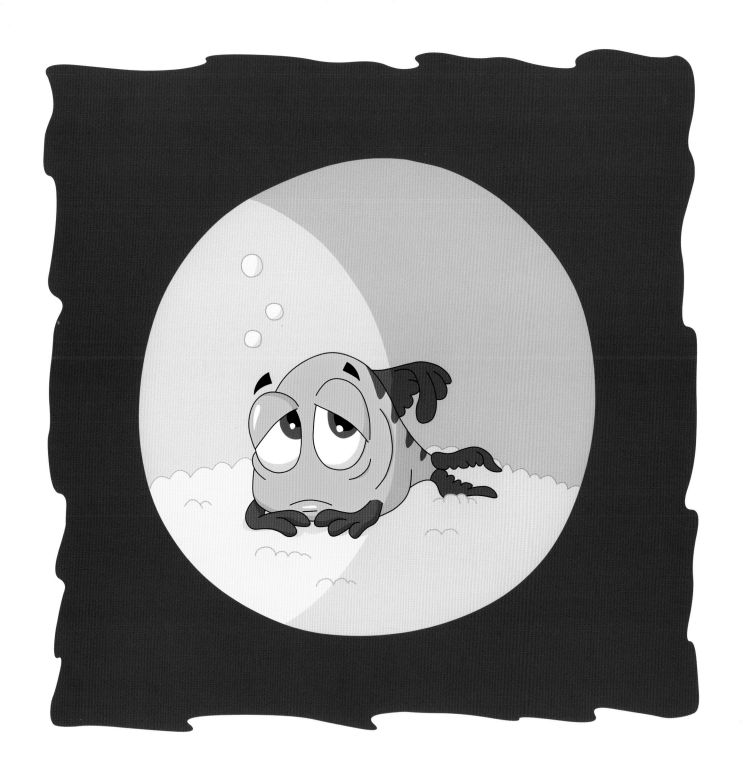

I only want to be a fish if I can eat fruit, he thought.

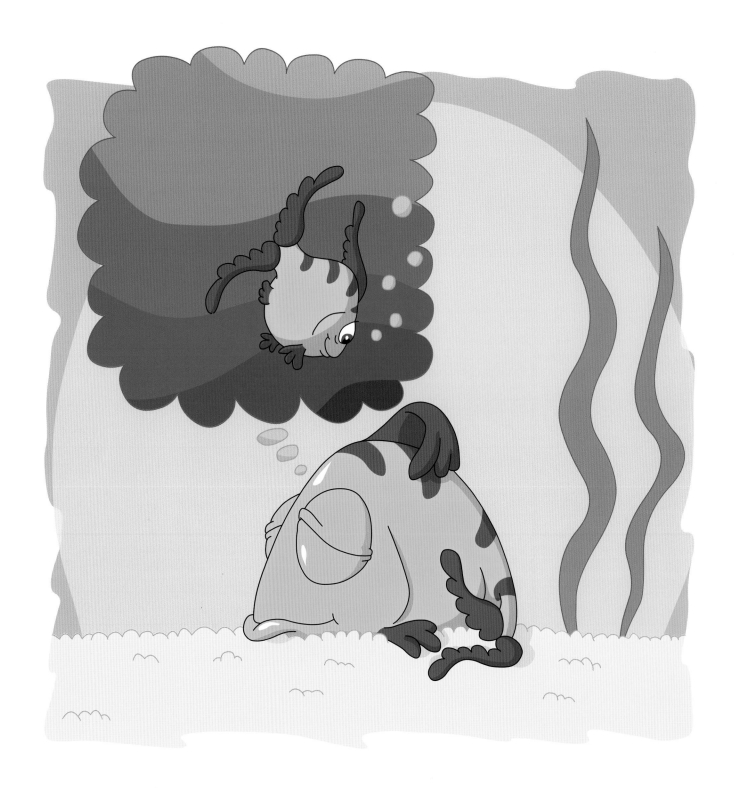

His eyes grew heavy as he fell fast asleep.
As he began to dream, he saw himself swimming
toward the bottom of the deep blue sea.

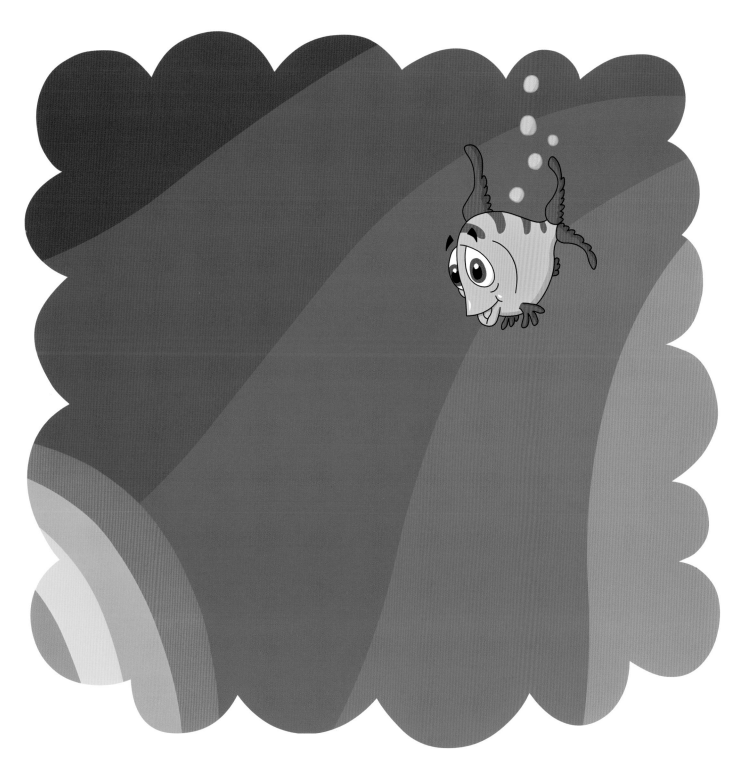

Halfway down, he stopped in amazement.
What's that? he wondered.
He blinked a few times and hurried to the bottom.

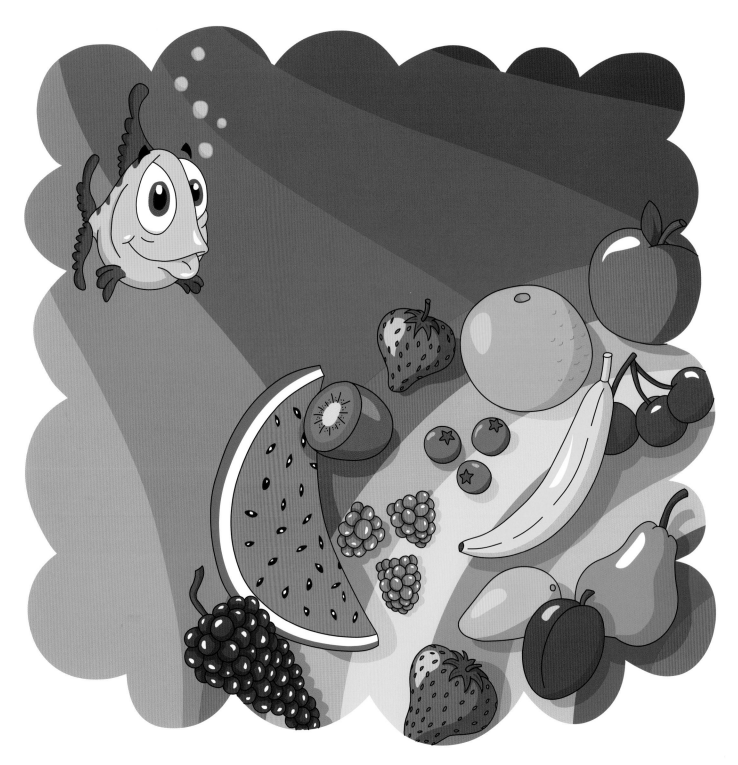

His eyes grew very large as he approached
a beautiful Rainbow Water Forest
filled with bright and colorful fruits.

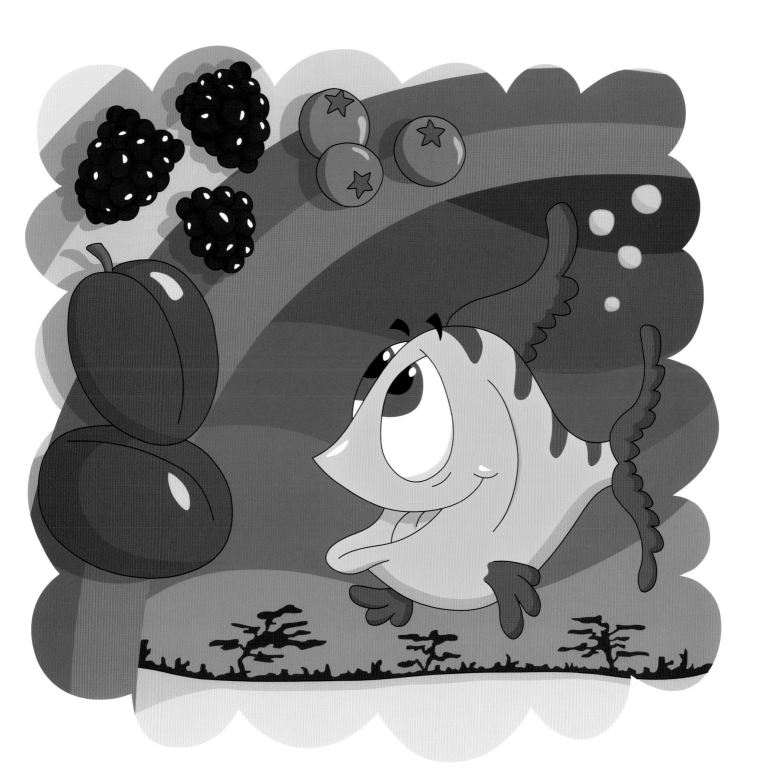

Theo saw blueberries, black raspberries and purple plums.

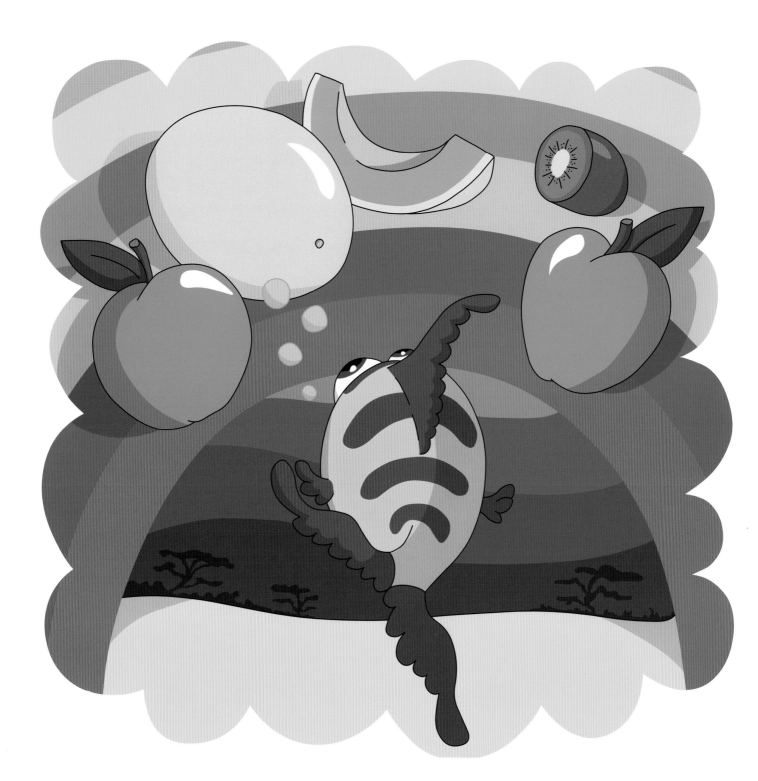

He discovered green honeydew melons,
kiwis and green apples.

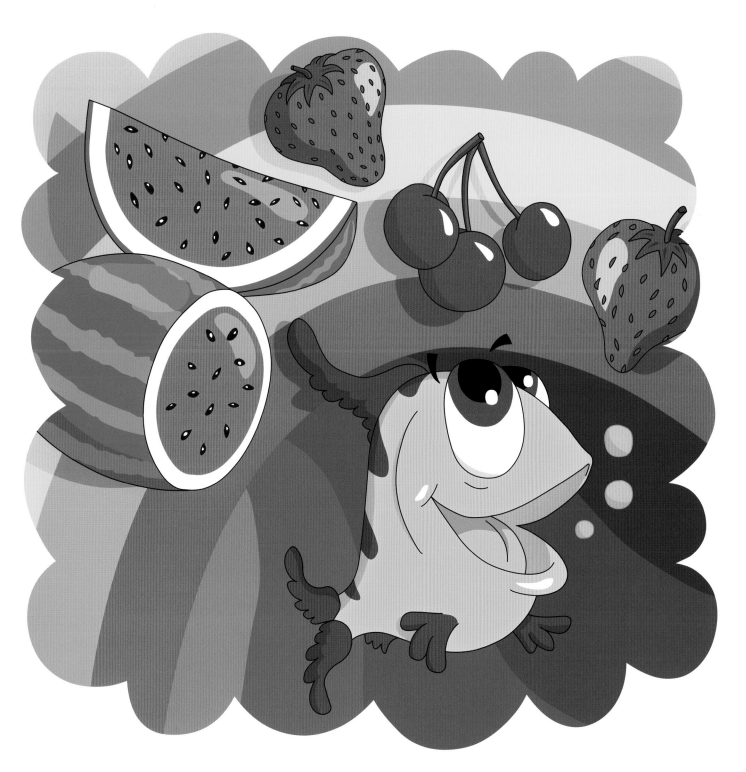

He was excited about the red watermelons,
strawberries and red cherries.

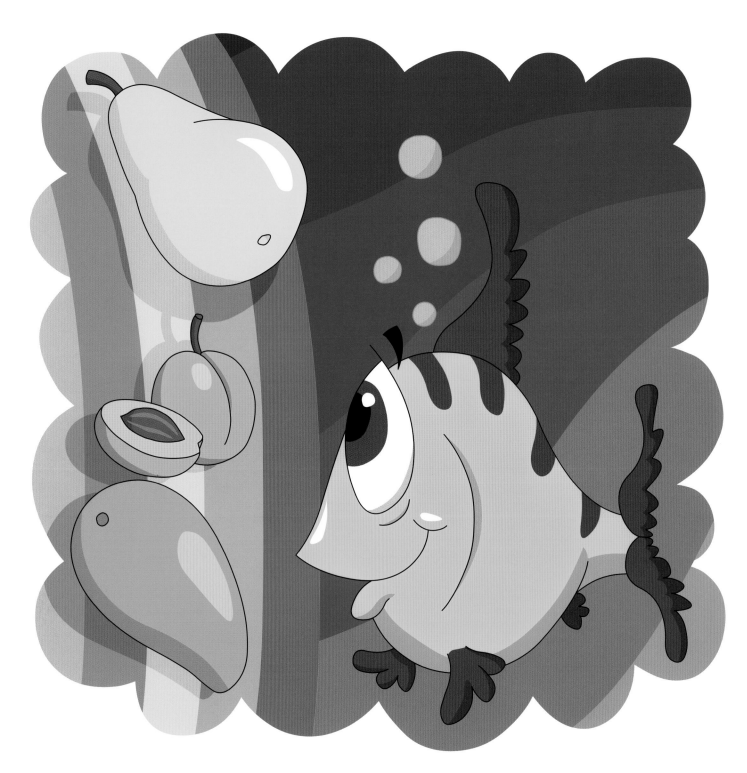

He was curious about the yellow pears,
apricots and mangos.

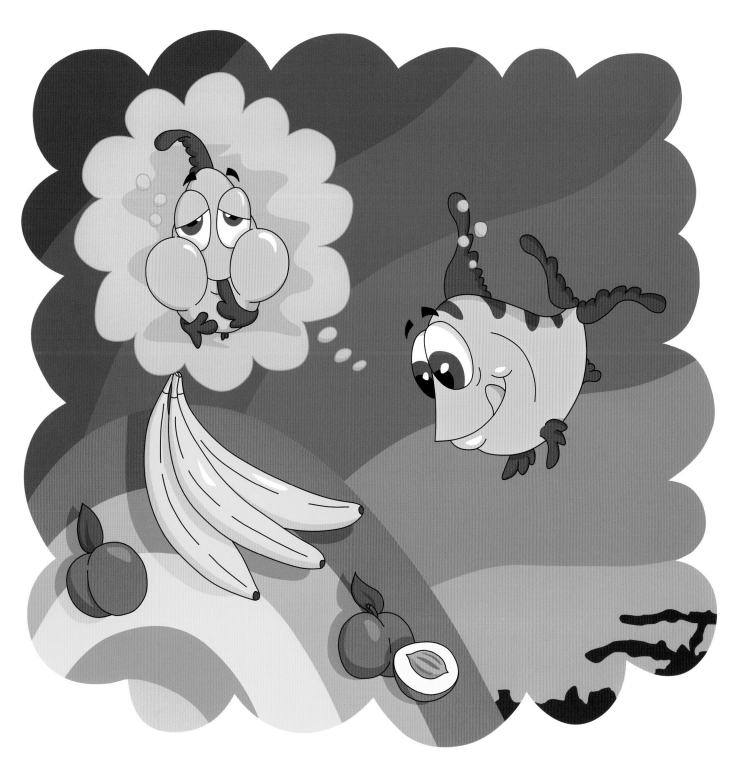

And he couldn't wait to try the bananas
and white peaches.

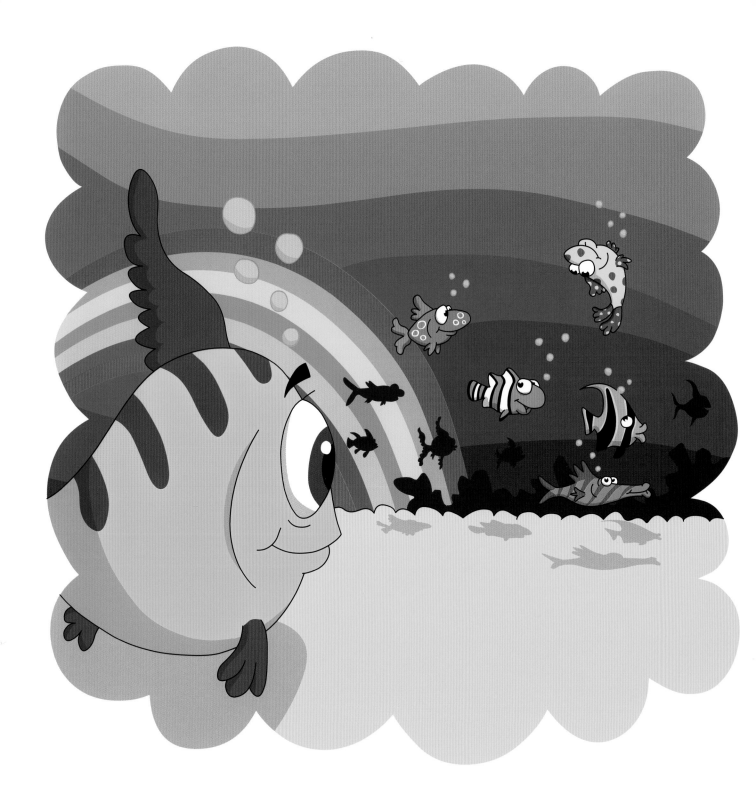

He also saw other fish in the Rainbow Water Forest. They were as colorful as the fruits. Theo was amazed at how beautiful and graceful the other fish appeared.

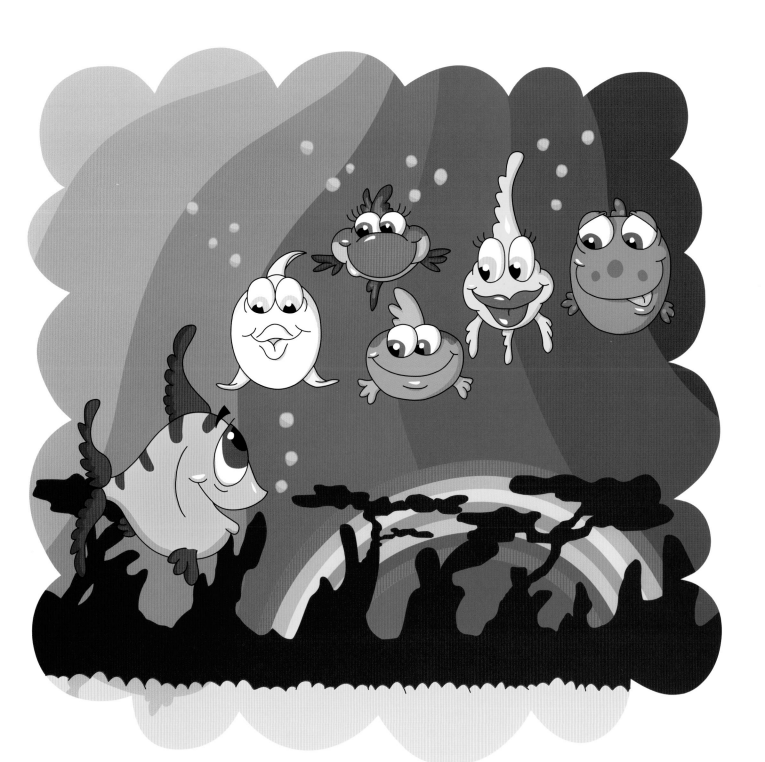

At that moment, five of the brightest
fish swam closer to him.
"You are all so beautiful," he said.

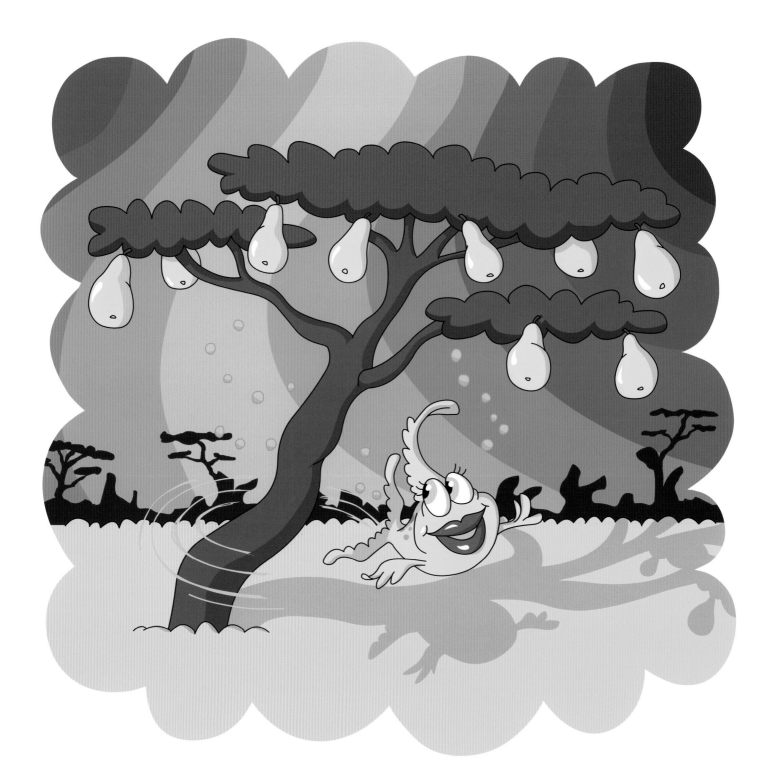

"That's because we eat fruit,"
said the twinkling yellow fish
as she danced around the pear tree.

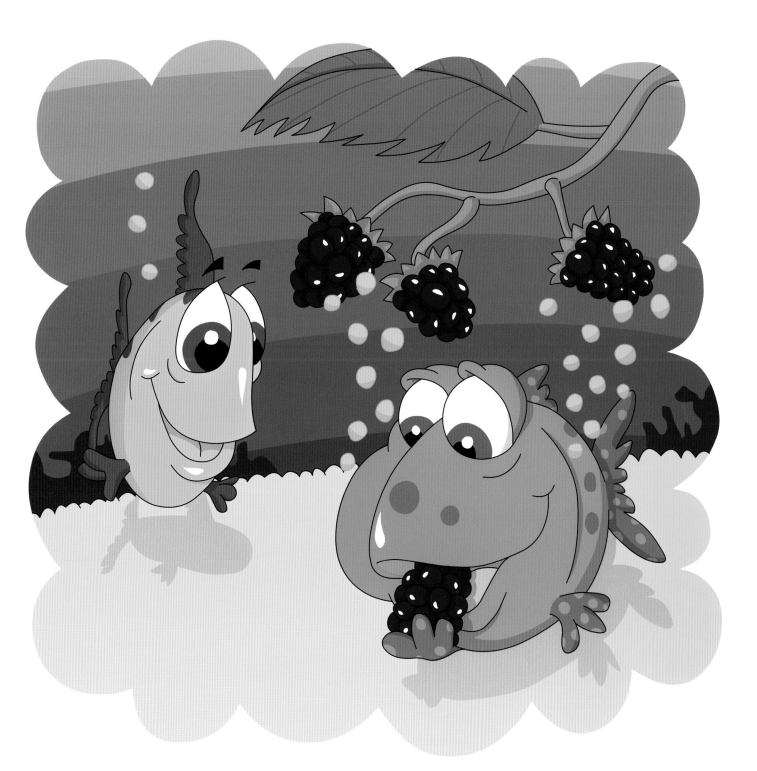

"Really?" asked Theo.
"Absolutely," said the sparkling blue fish.
"And look how strong my gills are!" He took one very
deep breath, then swallowed a black raspberry.

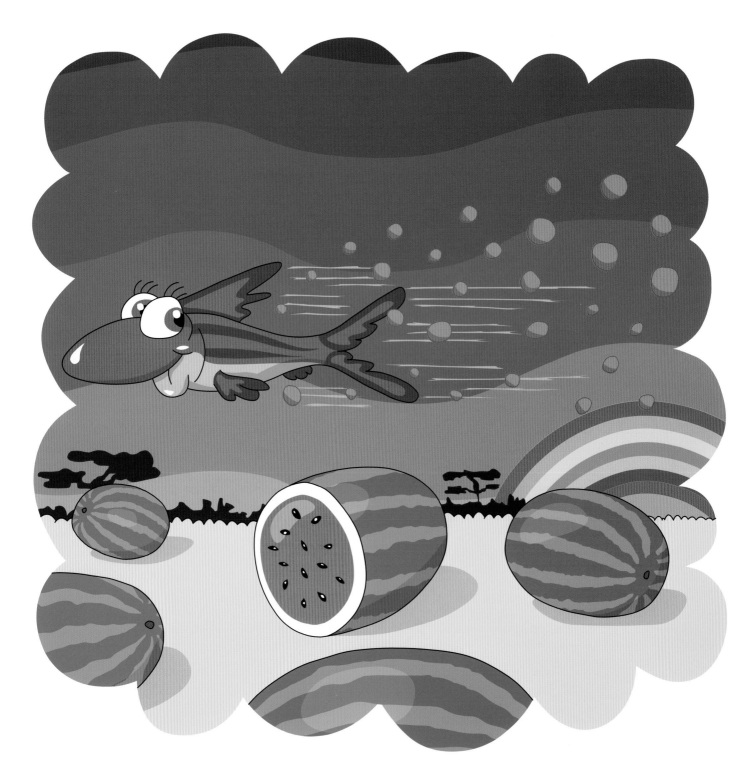

"Watch how fast I can swim!"
said the shimmering red fish.
She raced across the watermelon patch,
leaving red bubbles behind her.

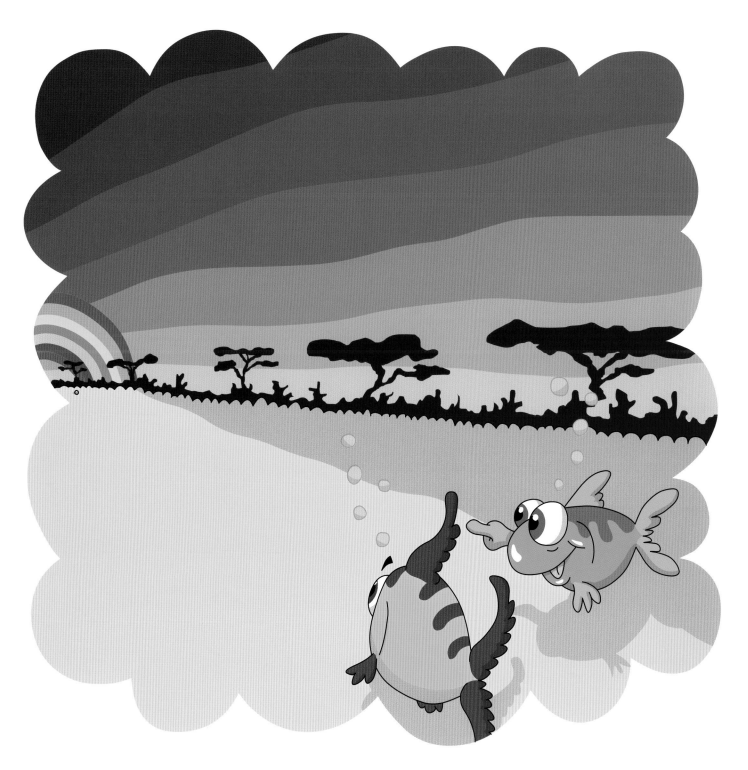

"I can see for miles!"
said the shiny green fish
as he pointed to a green grape
on the other side of the forest.

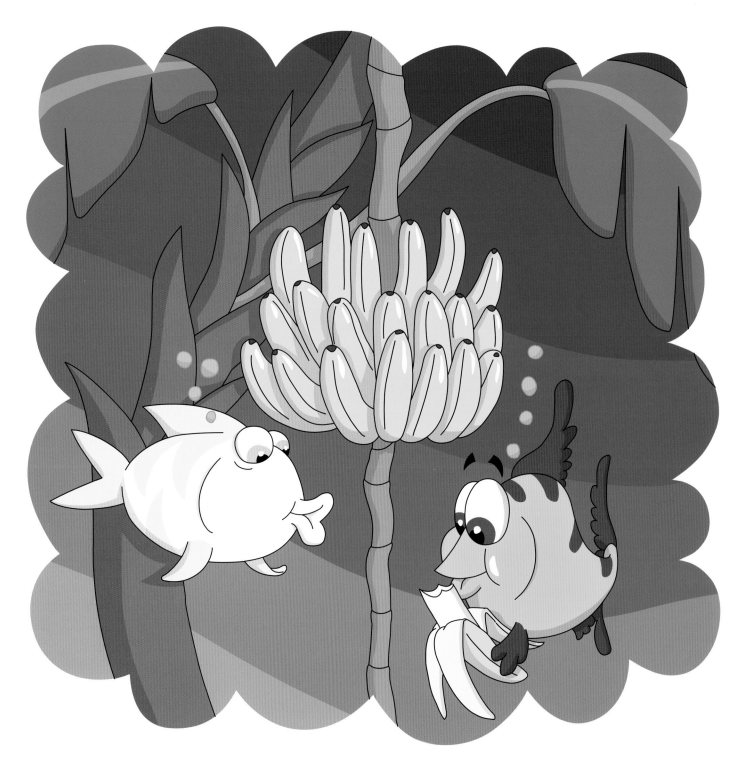

"I love bananas," said the glowing white fish.
Before Theo could spot the bananas,
the white fish grabbed one for him to taste.
"Delicious! I love bananas too!" said Theo.

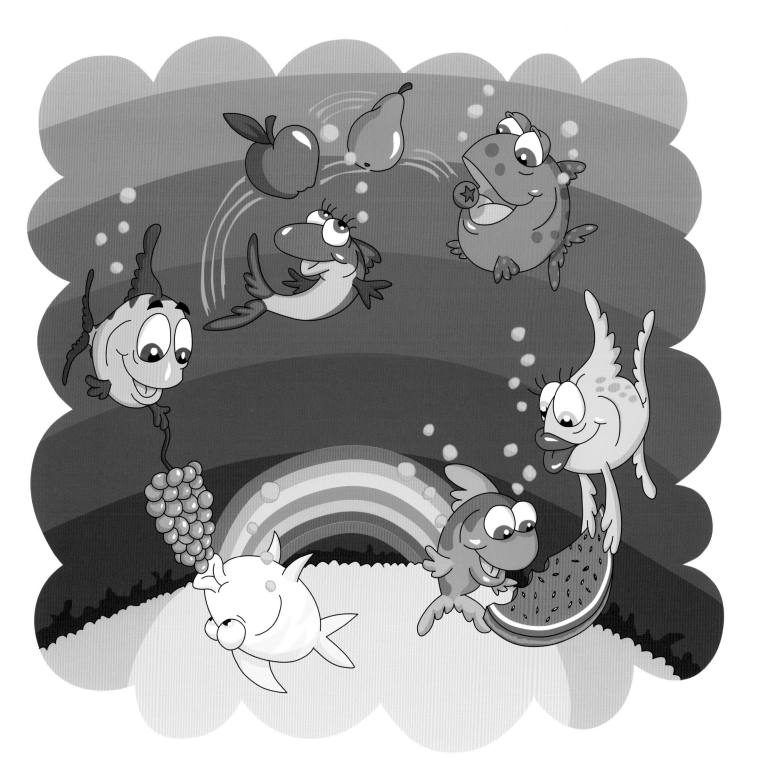

For the next several hours, Theo and his five new friends played and laughed and tasted all the wonderful fruits in the Rainbow Water Forest.

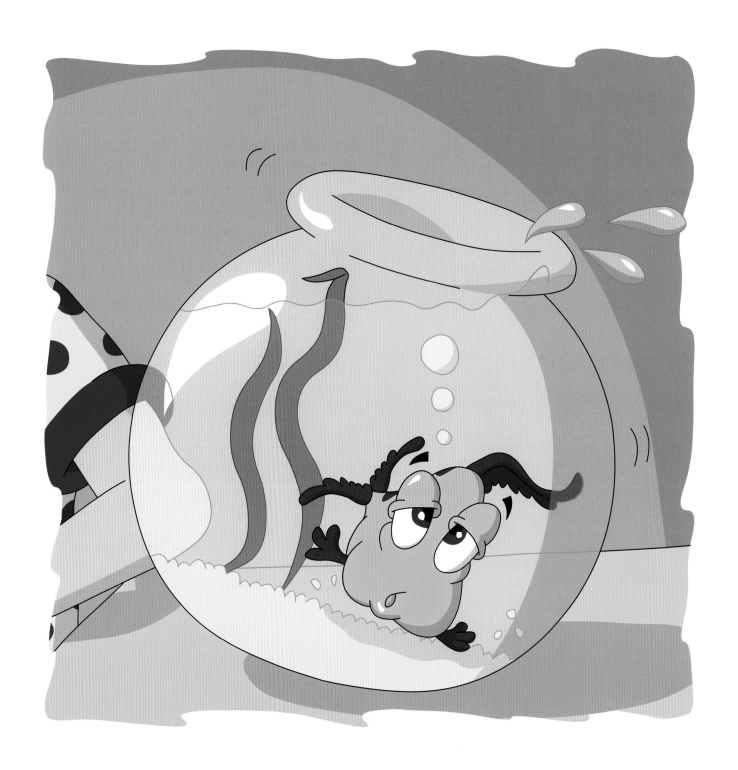

Suddenly, one of the children bumped the
fish bowl and Theo woke up. He shook his tail
and realized he was back home.

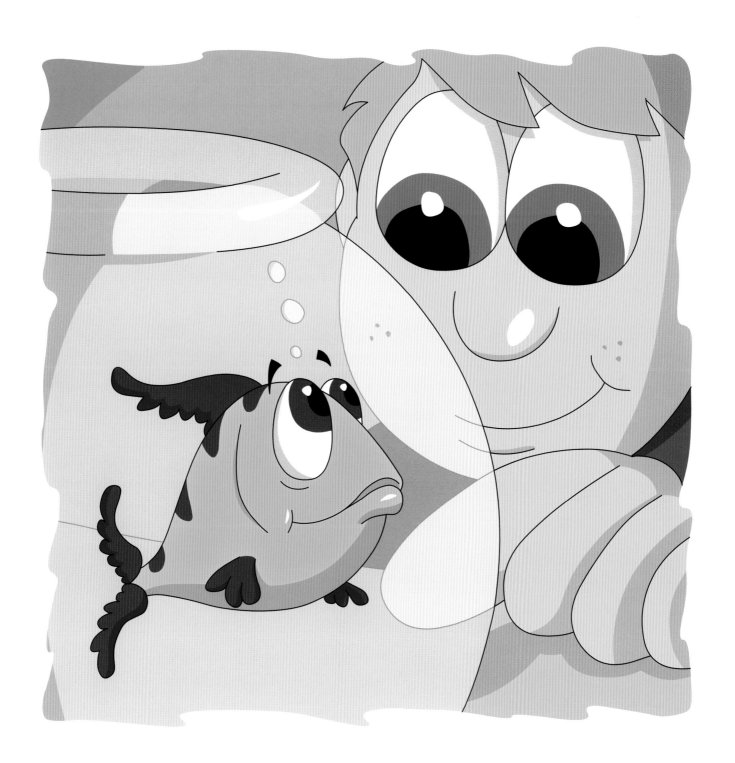

As he looked around, he noticed one of the little boys staring at the bottom of his bowl.

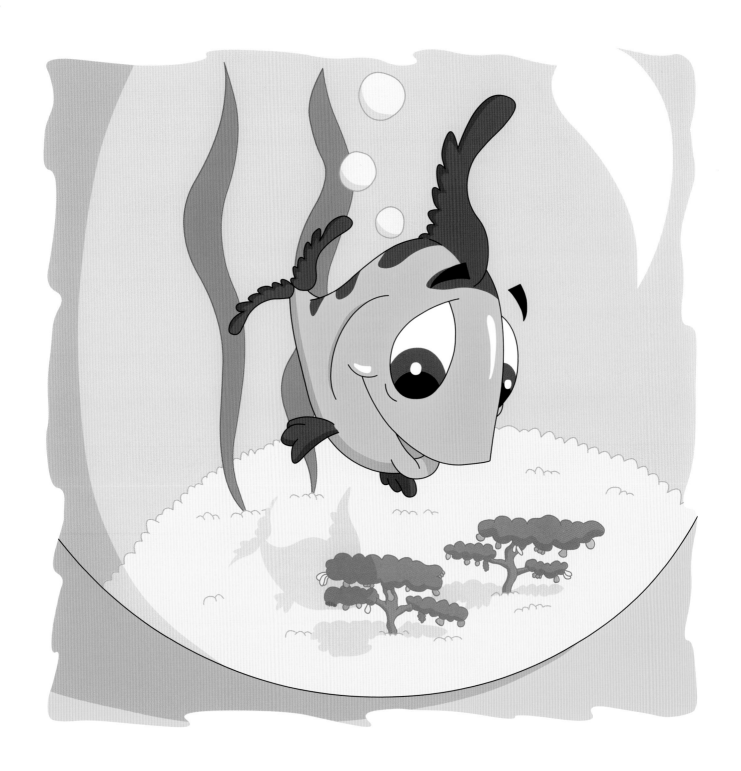

Theo looked down and saw two little trees
growing right up from the bottom. Each tree
held small, colorful pieces of fruit.

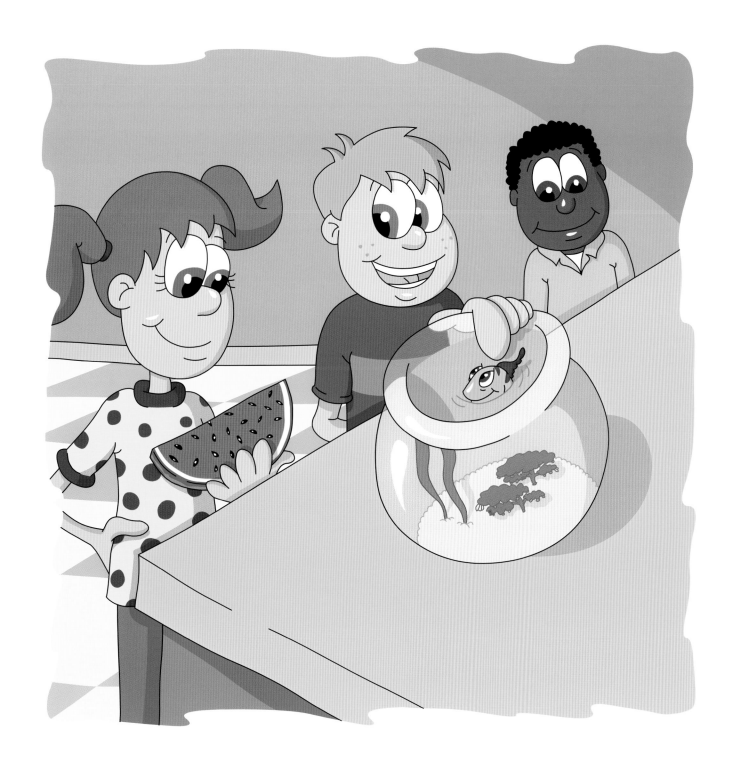

Amazed, the boy said,
"I wish I was a fish, so I could eat those fruits."

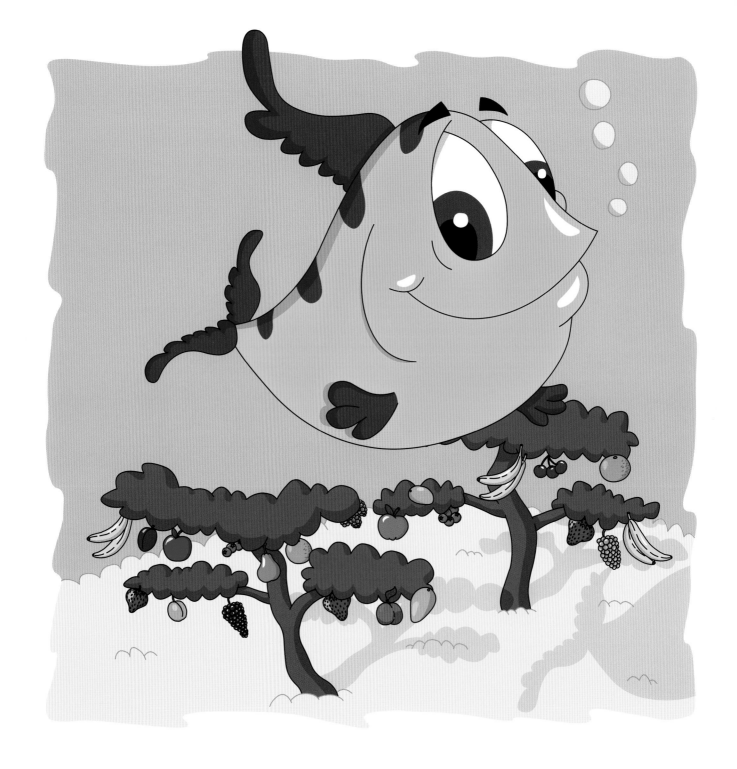

Theo smiled and swam around his fish bowl, happy that he was a fish, a fish who could eat fruit.

Fruits and Veggies Keep My Body Healthy

Whole, Fresh, Raw, Ripe, Organic

Why Should Kids Eat A Rainbow of Colors?

Add more YELLOW and ORANGE fruits and veggies to help keep your:

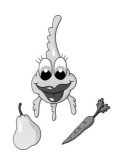

- Heart strong
- Vision clear
- A healthy immune system
- A lower risk of some cancers

Include more BLUE and PURPLE fruits and veggies to help keep your:

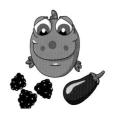

- Body healthy as it grows
- Memory sharp
- Urinary tract healthy
- A lower risk of some cancers

Add more RED fruits and veggies to help keep your:

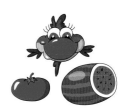

- Heart strong
- Memory sharp
- Urinary tract healthy
- A lower risk of some cancers

Include more GREEN fruits and veggies to help keep your:

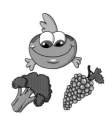

- Bones and teeth strong
- Vision clear
- A lower risk of some cancers

Add more WHITE fruits and veggies to help keep your:

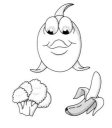

- Heart strong
- Maintain cholesterol levels that are already healthy
- A lower risk of some cancers

Source: National Cancer Institute and the Produce for Better Health Foundation

Matching Game

Match the color of each fruit and veggie to the color on the body.
Use the Color Key at the bottom to understand how the colors of fruits and veggies keep my body healthy.

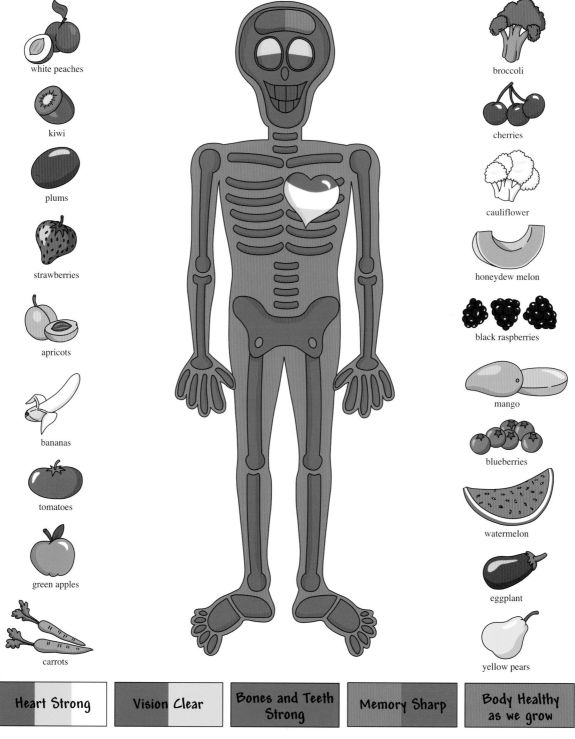

white peaches

kiwi

plums

strawberries

apricots

bananas

tomatoes

green apples

carrots

broccoli

cherries

cauliflower

honeydew melon

black raspberries

mango

blueberries

watermelon

eggplant

yellow pears

Heart Strong | Vision Clear | Bones and Teeth Strong | Memory Sharp | Body Healthy as we grow

*Note: Yellow and orange fruits and veggies have same health benefits; purple and blue fruits and veggies also have same health benefits.

15 Ways to Get Kids To Eat More Fruits and Vegetables

1. Green smoothies- a delicious blend of fruits and green leafy veggies; See recipes on next page.

2. Be a good role model. Eat and enjoy a variety of fruit and veggies yourself.

3. Have a bowl of fruit on the kitchen table for a quick, easy snack.

4. Always have freshly cut veggie sticks in the refrigerator.

5. Try many times — fifteen or more — to get your kids to eat their veggies. Don't give up.

6. Let your kids help choose fresh veggies when you're shopping.

7. Get your kids involved in fruit, veggie and salad preparation. They are more likely to eat something they helped make. Have them peel bananas, shuck corn, or scoop watermelon into balls.

8. Add veggies to the foods your kids already like.

9. Try different textures of fruits. For example, bananas are smooth and creamy, apples are crunchy, and oranges are juicy.

10. Great snack idea - In a 12-cup muffin pan, cut up small pieces of fruits and veggies and place them in each cup. Leave the muffin pan out all day for kids to snack on.

11. Make fancy shapes - use a melon baller, apple slicer, or cookie cutter. For example, pick a shape and introduce everything that is circle shaped - slices of cucumber, round slices of carrot, apple rings, cherries, strawberries, melon balls. The next day, cube everything and challenge your kids to try squares of fruit and veggies - do they taste the same?

12. Decorate plates or serving dishes with fruit slices.

13. Make fruit kabobs using pineapple chunks, bananas, grapes, and berries.

14. Freeze grapes, bananas and mango wedges for a refreshing and cool treat.

15. Peanut Butter Flowers - Place a tablespoon of peanut butter in center of plate. Slice carrots or celery thinly and place the slices in a circular pattern to create peanut butter "flowers".

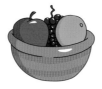

Green Smoothie recipes
A blend of fresh fruits and green veggies

Green smoothies are a wonderful way to include more fresh green leafy veggies into your kid's diet. It tastes just like a fruit smoothie only its green. Enjoy!

Spinach Surprise

1-½ cups spinach
1 banana
1 yellow apple
water

Romaine Rush

6 large pieces romaine lettuce
2 red apples
1 stalk celery
water

Dandelion Delight

1-1/2 cups dandelion greens
1 green apple
1 banana
1 stalk celery
water

Kale Kiss

1 cup dinosaur (lacinato) Kale
(cut out stems)
1 banana
1 cup strawberries
water

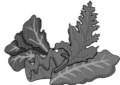

Instructions:

1. Put enough water in blender to cover the blade.

2. Wash and cut up fresh or frozen fruit and blend with the water.

3. Wash and cut up fresh veggies and add to blender until smooth consistency.

4. Add more water for thinner consistency.

5. Pour into a glass and drink, or pour into a bowl and eat it with a spoon.

Be creative, make your own smoothies. Include your kids.
Best greens to use include romaine lettuce, kale, spinach, chard,
celery, parsley, dandelion greens, Boston lettuce, frisee lettuce.
Best fruits to use include all apples, pears, strawberries, pineapple,
blueberries, bananas, mango, kiwi, raspberries.